MALE KEGEL EXERCISES FOR NOVICES

A STEP BY STEP GUIDE FOE EXERCISES FOR THE MALE KEGEL

KYLE NEAL

Table of Contents

CHAPTER ONE

Exercises for the Male Kegel

What exactly are Kegel exercises?

To strengthen your pelvic floor muscles, you can perform kegel exercises. Your bladder and bowels are controlled by these muscles. It also aids in the development of erections.

There are a number of muscles and tissues that run from your tailbone to your pubic bone. Your bladder and bowel are supported by your muscles. In order for urine (pee) and feces (poop) to exit your body, they must pass through the muscles and tissues of the pelvic floor, which includes the urethra.

Do men do Kegel exercises for whatever reason?

Kegel exercises can be helpful for men who have specific health or sexual health issues. You may benefit from these exercises:

As a result, incontinence can be alleviated

• Treat pain and swelling in the prostate caused by prostatitis and BPH (BPH).

• Improved orgasm sensation and better control of ejaculation can increase your sexual pleasure.

Your muscles must be identified prior to beginning Kegel exercises. To perform a proper Kegel exercise, you must locate and flex three muscles.

Using the bulbocavernosus (BC) muscle, you push blood into the penis and squeeze urine and semen out of your urethra and penis.

The pubococcygeus (PC) muscle is another. This muscle helps you urinate and defecate, and it contracts during sex. Your lower organs are supported by it.

• The third muscle is the iliococcygeus muscle (IC), which supports your organs and aids in the repositioning of your anus after you urinate.

When performing Kegel exercises, the BC muscle does the bulk of the work, with the other two assisting only slightly. When you're peeing, you can find this muscle by halting the flow of urine.

Your PC muscle can be felt if you try to shorten your penis by attempting to draw your penis toward your body. It's possible that you'll experience an upward pull on your scrotum.

Find your IC muscle by mimicking a movement you would make if you were trying to hold in your diarrhea or prevent yourself from passing gas.

Your genital muscles contract and relax.

CHAPTER TWO

If you're going to start an exercise program, you should take baby steps at first.

• Kegel exercises can be done anywhere, but laying or sitting on your bed is a good place to start.

For about five seconds, squeeze your pelvic floor muscles. Counting aloud can help you relax and avoid holding your breath. Then take a five-second break.

Make a total of 10 repetitions in a row. Do three sessions a day, if possible. Stopping when you're tired is a good idea.

• When performing Kegel exercises, you should not feel any discomfort. Doing them incorrectly may be the source of your discomfort. Now is the time to consult with your doctor or other healthcare professional. As a physical therapist, they may have suggestions for how you can improve your pelvic floor exercises technique or provide you with a physical therapy program that includes biofeedback.

To avoid pain and ensure proper muscle function, it's critical to master the art of relaxing your pelvic floor muscles.

The benefits of male Kegel exercises

Kegel exercises can improve bladder and bowel health, as well as your sex life. Prostate cancer patients preparing for surgery may benefit from these exercises as well.

Who should not do Kegel exercises?

If you learn how to relax and strengthen your kegel muscles, you won't injure yourself. You should not overdo it with Kegel exercises. In addition, attempting to stop your urine from flowing should be avoided at all costs.

If you have a urinary catheter in place, avoid doing Kegel exercises.

How long will it take before you notice a change in your body?

Kegel exercises can take up to six weeks before you start to see any real progress. To keep reaping their rewards, it's imperative that you incorporate them into your daily routine.

Cleveland Clinic issued a statement on the matter

The muscles in your pelvic floor require regular exercise in order to maintain their strength. You can ask your doctor for advice on how to do Kegel exercises for your pelvic floor muscles. Performing these exercises may help you stop leaking urine or feces, as well as improve your sexual performance and enjoyment.. It may be awkward to discuss, but there are ways to improve these situations. Making your life more pleasurable is worth the effort.

Kegel Exercises: A Quick and Easy Guide

Make sure your bladder is empty before beginning your Kegel exercises.

Begin by taking the following steps:

To begin, squeeze your pelvic floor muscles for five seconds at a time. The best way to do this is to imagine yourself bringing your genitals in and lifting them up.

Make sure you don't hold your breath as you do this. Holding

Ayour breath can be relieved by counting aloud.

Relax your muscles for 5 seconds after holding for 5 seconds.

3. Perform this procedure ten times, at least three times daily.

During this exercise, your pelvic floor muscles may become fatigued. If this happens, stop and come back to it at a later time.

When performing this exercise, avoid using the muscles in your stomach, legs, or buttocks. You won't be able to regain control of your bladder or improve your sexual health by working these muscles.

Increase the amount of time you hold and rest your pelvic floor muscles as you continue to practice these exercises. Slowly increase the time each week by 5 seconds. Then rest for a full 10 seconds before repeating this process.

CHAPTER THREE

Kegel Exercises: A Quick and Easy Guide

Make sure your bladder is empty before beginning your Kegel exercises.

Begin by taking the following steps:

To begin, squeeze your pelvic floor muscles for five seconds at a time. The best way to do this is to imagine yourself bringing your genitals in and lifting them up.

Make sure you don't hold your breath as you do this. Holding your breath can be relieved by counting aloud.

Relax your muscles for 5 seconds after holding for 5 seconds.

3. Perform this procedure ten times, at least three times daily.

During this exercise, your pelvic floor muscles may become fatigued. If this happens, stop and come back to it at a later time.

When performing this exercise, avoid using the muscles in your stomach, legs, or buttocks. You won't be able to regain control of your bladder or improve your sexual health by working these muscles.

Increase the amount of time you hold and rest your pelvic floor muscles as you continue to practice these exercises. Slowly increase the time each week by 5 seconds. Then rest for a full

10 seconds before repeating this process.

Pain and Kegel exercises

Should kegel exercises hurt? They're enjoyable and soothing for the majority of people. Kegel exercises can be uncomfortable if you use the wrong muscles.

• If you experience pain in your back or stomach after performing Kegel exercises, it's possible that you're using muscles other than the ones in your pelvic floor.

A headache may be caused by tightening and holding your chest muscles while doing Kegel exercises.

When to Contact Your Doctor

If you are experiencing any of the following:

- If you're concerned about your bowel, bladder, or sexual health.

-

- Are you unable to feel the muscles in your pelvic floor?

- Be unable to perform Kegel exercises because of pain.

Kegel exercises are challenging for you.

- You're experiencing discomfort in your lower abdomen.

• Seeking a recommendation for a pelvic health physical therapist.

Do Kegel exercises for men need to be done on a regular basis?

Push-ups and sit-ups are common exercises for men. But only a small percentage of them are familiar with Kegel exercises. Many doctors recommend incorporating these into one's daily routine, which is a shame.

When it comes to Kegel exercises, there is no magic number of sets that one should perform in a day. Men, on the other hand, should perform two sets of Kegel exercises every day at the very least. First thing in the morning and last thing at night are the best times for men to exercise. Ten to thirty contractions and relaxation exercises are included in each session. Ten seconds of contraction and five seconds of relaxation should be allotted for each exercise. Once a man has mastered these, he can perform them in a variety of ways. He can perform a third of the exercises while lying down, a third while sitting, and a third while standing, out of the 10-30 total. Counting out loud is a great way to get started, and many men are pleasantly surprised by how naturally they can perform the exercises they initially found difficult.

For men undergoing prostate surgery, whether for cancer of the prostate requiring radical prostatectomy (complete removal of the prostate) or for BPH requiring transurethral resection of the prostate, this is of the utmost importance. Both of these procedures reduce the bladder's resistance, which can lead to postoperative incontinence. The following image shows how the anatomical changes reduce the resistance of the bladder outlet. To that end, Kegel exercises can assist in building a strong pelvic floor and sphincter. The Kegel exercises should begin well in advance of surgery and continue for a few weeks following the procedure.

Premature Ejaculation and Erectile Dysfunction (ED) Kegel Exercises

If you can't get or keep an erection, you're suffering from "erectile dysfunction" (ED). Erectile dysfunction affects an estimated 18 million men in the United States, a number that rises with increasing age. It's estimated that one in three men will suffer from an ED at some point in their lives.

Early release of semen in sexual intercourse is referred to as premature ejaculation. A man's self-esteem and sexual relationships can be negatively affected by premature ejaculation, even though it is not a medical condition.

Many doctors now believe that one's overall health and one's sexual well-being go hand in hand. 44 percent of men who have erectile dysfunction are affected by health complications like diabetes and hypertension, according to a recent study (high blood pressure).

CHAPTER FOUR

Many of these problems can be treated without resorting to expensive drugs or time-consuming treatments. The core and pelvic area of the body can be strengthened through a variety of exercises, including Kegel exercises.

Premature ejaculation can be addressed by strengthening the muscles surrounding and supporting the genital area, which helps the penis maintain an erection.

Improve erection and prevent premature ejaculation with kegel exercises.

Erectile dysfunction should be treated with kegel exercises, or pelvic exercises, as the first line of treatment. An erection is activated by the ischiocavernosus and bulbocavernosus muscles in the pelvic area that surround the penis. These muscles can be strengthened by performing the exercises listed below.

Squeezing Your Back on the Floor

Laying on your back, hands flat on the floor, and knees bent and pointing upwards is an excellent place to begin this exercise.

Hold your penis in this position for five seconds before releasing it.

To stop a bowel movement, squeeze your anus muscles and hold them for five seconds before releasing them.

4. Repeat steps two and three, eight to ten times, and perform

three to five sets of three to five repetitions each.

Squeezing Your Side on the Floor

1. Lie on your side on the floor.

Place a pillow between your knees to help alleviate pain. Make sure your legs can be separated on the pillow.

Hold your legs together for five seconds, then let go.

Repeat step three eight to ten times, and complete three to five sets of each.

Squeezing into a Chair Makes You Feel Smaller.

Sit down in a chair and find a comfortable position.

If you can't stop the urine from leaking from your penis, squeeze it for five seconds and then let go.

Step 2 should be repeated eight to ten times, and then three to five sets should be completed.

The squeezing technique can be tested by trying to halt the flow of urine for a few seconds. You're doing it correctly if you're able to.

Squeeze and hold the different pelvic muscles for longer as your body gets used to the exercises. Doing more sets or repetitions of an exercise is also an option.

Keep these tips in mind while performing these exercises:

Avoid suffocating yourself

• Instead of pushing down, tighten your pelvic muscles as if you were trying to lift something.

Relax your stomach muscles as much as possible.

Your pelvic floor muscles should be relaxed between squeezes to prevent injury.

With consistent daily exercise, most men begin to see positive changes after about a month of regular training. By the end of the month, you should be able to hold the squeezes for 10 seconds and perform eight to 10 sets of eight to ten repetitions.

Precautions to Be Taken

Exercises should not cause any discomfort at all. If you feel any pain, immediately stop the exercises and seek medical attention.

THE END

www.ingramcontent.com/pod-product-compliance
Lightning Source LLC
Chambersburg PA
CBHW051406150726
48000CB00003B/1357